Lilly in the Valley: Unapologetically

By Lillie Marie

Contents

Introduction

Oftentimes women turn the other cheek in marriage for the sake of the marriage itself. She knows better and wants better but second-guesses her strength, power, and purpose. When does that woman matter? When do you put yourself first? When do you live your life unapologetically?

As women, wives, and mothers, we often lose ourselves in all that comes with these responsibilities: the house duties, the husband responsibilities, the children. The reality is that most of us create our own little bubbles of comfort. But when do you choose self? When do you say enough is enough?

For me, it was when he packed his stuff and left us.

This is my story! A story of a married woman who was comfortable and fulfilled—or so she thought! It wasn't until that fateful night when my husband and the father of our children walked away that the transformation occurred. What transformation, you might be asking? The one that took me from married woman to single mom to a broken version of myself to who I now know as Lillie—or more importantly—Lilly of the Valley!

Walk with me on this journey of shock, enlightenment, hardship, and triumph. Ultimately, I hope to inspire you to view your life through a new lens and see your value as God sees you.

"And He said to me, 'My grace is sufficient for you, for My strength is made perfect in weakness.' Therefore, most gladly I will rather boast in my infirmities, that the power of Christ may rest upon me." II Corinthians 12:9 NKJV

All hell broke loose on November 14th, 2020.

My girls, Laylah and Lyric, had a cotillion ball to attend. It was a very joyous event. The girls looked beautiful, and we took many memorable family photos as a smiling, seemingly happy family unit.

Until we arrived home….then my husband decided to pack all of his stuff and leave!

I guess he had been thinking about it for some time and chose that moment to pull the trigger.

Confused. Shocked. Uncertain.

But most importantly, I wasn't going to stop him!

We had built a good life together and had a picture-perfect family, doing everything together. However, I knew that if this was not good for him, I did not want to hold him back from being a great version of himself. I would not stand in his way, and if this was what it would take for him to feel, achieve, or be what he wanted, I would let him go.

Of course, we had arguments over the nearly nine years of our marriage. We had disagreements like many married couples have, but nothing to the magnitude of divorce in my eyes. I can only speak for myself anyway.

When he returned to our family home the following day to pick up the rest of his belongings, I was prepared with a separation agreement which I had him sign.

Tension was high, and tempers were even higher. At this point, egos were still in the way, so it was difficult to comprehend that we would go through with a divorce.

The girls watched with pain in their hearts as mommy and daddy argued. We did not even try to hide anything from them, and I later found them crying in their beds. They were certainly as confused as I was, even maybe more so.

My husband was the breadwinner for our family, so our lives quickly began to change as he steadily pulled back month after month on the support he provided us; first, the car insurance, then the electric bill, then the car note. Every time I felt I was getting on my feet, bringing in a steady flow of income, he would pull the rug out from under me again, setting the girls and me back financially and, frankly, emotionally.

Each month I acquired a new burden, a new responsibility. Not only were we missing his physical presence in the home, but now all of our finances were also walking out the door. As the months passed, reality started to hit my girls, and they would cry every night. They loved their father and called him often but quickly learned he was pulling away from them too. He would either not answer his phone or reach out to them. He would peek in with them every now and then, but not enough to be a consistent parent in their lives.

I did not understand. This was not the person I had fallen in love with and married. He was showing a side of himself that I was not comfortable with. He was the kind of guy women would say to, "Your mama raised you right." Knowing this guy was not who I thought he was was a blow to me. He was nothing compared to what I saw him as. That type of guy wouldn't ruin his household for a fling if that were the case. That type of guy wouldn't destroy his family on a whim.

In April 2021, when he tried to reconcile and come back into the home, I was not having it. This man who I thought would always protect, love, and honor me was no longer the man trying to get back into our lives. As a woman raising two young girls, I knew I had to protect myself and them. I was moving cautiously, not in fear of him per se but knowing that when people are under a lot of stress or going through difficult times, they may be capable of anything.

I knew that allowing him to return would come at a cost, whether now or in the future. Would it have been my sacrifice? Would I have put my daughters' health and well-being in jeopardy? Would I have jeopardized my dignity by retaliating or harboring unforgiveness? At this point, the structure of our home had changed. All of the things we had done together, the foundation on which we were raising our daughters had been shaken, and the responsibility for their care and well-being had been placed on my shoulders for all those months. I had to think about my children. Knowing that his return would probably be only temporary, I was unwilling to gamble with my sanity or incur additional hurt by allowing him back into our lives. No! I was going through with the divorce.

So, when he showed up one day and let himself into my home with the key he still had, I knew what I had to do. As he tried to explain, I stood firm. "We were having a hard time, not seeing eye to eye," he said. "This was the best decision for me." Maybe that was the best decision for him, but when it comes to marriage and family, I do not see how walking away and calling it quits benefits anyone. It wasn't anger that I felt toward him at this point. I remained calm as I explained to him the disappointment and shock that surged through me of his neglect for us and our family. I had been with this man I loved since I was 19, and we had two beautiful children. He was my everything! Until then.

I calmly instructed him to leave my key alongside the garage door opener on the table. As I walked away, I saw the light go out in his eyes, and he stayed there for what seemed like an hour or so. Finally, sitting there on my couch, I saw the realization come over him that he had lost me.

We had counseling years before when he cheated on me, and during that session, I told him that if he ever cheated on me again, I would leave him. There was not going to be a second chance. Although I did not have confirmation that another woman was involved this time, as a woman, I just knew, and I had to follow through with my word. I was determined to push forward with the divorce.

I could understand how relationships change in marriage, but I could not fathom how a person so committed to being a hands-on father to his children suddenly avoids them as if they don't exist. I had never experienced this with anyone I knew, so I was dumbfounded about how he could just go cold turkey on his daughters. Who was this person?

At the time, Laylah and Lyric were eight and ten, too young to understand what was going on. What they had always known as their insular family had been ripped apart. What could I do but give them every opportunity to navigate this mess? So we went to counseling. I also knew God would pull us through and had to rely on my strong faith. We talked a lot, and I was open with them about what was happening. I went from being a married woman in a dual-income household to a single mother with one income; this was not easy for any of us. I had to go into survival mode for all of our sake and began to thrive.

Until August 2021!

I received a text message that read, "Leave my wife alone before you end up dead or you lose your job." One of the few expenses I was responsible for while we were married was the cell phone bill. Once we pushed forward with the divorce, I had him give me back the phone I had been paying for. So, when this text came through, I knew it must have had something to do with a woman. The girls had been spending time with their dad, so I knew he had a new girlfriend. I also figured this was not the same woman he had cheated on me with but another man's wife. The reality of it all hit me like a ton of bricks!

I had been living with a stranger for all of those years. I had my suspicions about infidelity, so that was not a big surprise. It was the audacity effect. We had been through so much together, yet I did not know who this man was. My feelings were hurt, and I could not run from the fact that everything I knew about him was probably not true.

I had to be strong for the girls. Their daddy wasn't there, and they had witnessed him packing and leaving. They had called him, and he didn't answer. How was I going to shield them from their own hurt and devastation? I did not want them to grow up having unresolved issues. I didn't want them poisoned with my own bitterness. I had learned from my mother how to handle adult things when it came to children. She never badgered my father in front of me, only saying instead, "You will see when you get older." I knew the healthiness of not exposing children to too much and the value of talking openly to them if they wanted to talk about it. I did not want to paint him in a negative light in their eyes, yet I had to consider their feelings and how they would relate to men as they got older.

I was in survival mode and had been nurturing everything and everyone except myself. Yes, the girls had lost their father in a way, but I had lost my husband. When that text came in, the reality was too much to bear. I confronted him, and he denied everything, even insinuating that I had sent the text to *myself*. He never wanted to talk about what actually happened, denying me the closure I deserved. But I knew that I had been a good wife to him. The Lord knows I may not be perfect, but I tried to be perfect for *him*. And with this, and knowing that no man or woman on this earth could ever give me what God has already supplied, I was comfortable moving on with my life. I knew I had given everything to that marriage, but if that wasn't good enough for him, I was comfortable saying that I loved him enough to let him go. I also knew that I loved myself more and would not allow his misery to bring me stress, disease, or kill me in the process. I was able to walk away with a clear conscious because I knew I had given him the best that I could. If nothing else, I earned that 'R' in Mrs.

I did not want to become one of those women who said, just because I was married or had kids by this man, I want to be with him because we love each other and can fight through anything together. Metaphorically speaking, once he let my hand go, what was I supposed to do with that? No, he let it go. He packed his stuff and walked out the door. He left me there to deal with the depression. He left me there to deal with the anxiety. He left me there to deal with Laylah and Lyric. He left me there to deal with the bills. He walked away!!

Unfortunately, I see many women fall into this trap of false marriage. You can be married and still be miserable. You can be married and be a single parent, feeling alone. Just because you are married does not fix anything unless the other person is willing to fix it with you. If you are willing to stay in the ring with me, we can fight life together all day. But what should a person do if their partner steps out of that ring?

Well, you continue to fight because you have to! Marriage is supposed to be a selfless act if you are going to do it right. It has nothing to do with the kids or the husband/wife titles. I was so used to him doing everything. Now I'm not weak by far, but as his wife, I allowed him to handle things, and he supposedly loved to do that for his family. I let him be the man of the house. As a police officer, he upheld his duty to protect and serve, which includes his family. Before him, I had lived on my own, working two jobs to support myself. I was no stranger to working or managing things, but I got comfortable allowing him to.

So that's why I didn't understand the treatment my girls and I were now receiving from him. Maybe he was acting. On second thought, maybe it was a standard I had set that he wouldn't show me any other side than the one I wanted to see. It makes me wonder if this new man is the true *him*, but it wasn't *him* when he was connected to me.

I had a standard for how I expected to be treated, and I believe every woman should do that. We all should have high expectations of how we deserve to be treated by men, and there should be no exceptions. We teach our daughters to value themselves and to expect nothing less than what they deserve. Unfortunately, many women do not hold men accountable or are willing to accept less than being treated with respect, honor, and value. My husband may have been trying to live up to my expectations, but that might not have been who he was all along.

And I had to be okay with that. I realized that walking away from what was no longer feeding my growth was okay. I just didn't see it until it was presented to me in a life-changing way. It doesn't matter how long a relationship has lasted. The number of years is only of value if you both value them.

Today I see my ex-husband through a different lens. Everything happened so quickly that I didn't have time to check in to see how I felt. I had too much to worry about, making my girls' safety and security a priority over my own well-being and mental state. I knew that if I didn't take care of them, I could lose them to the world. I had to rely on my faith as my strength to get me through.

I refused to be the victim. As God says, I have always wanted to be victorious over it all. Although I wasn't expecting infidelity and divorce, it happened. Knowing that my story is already written, I know my life would have taken this path regardless of what I had done or expected from my marriage.

God only gives us what we can handle, so He equipped me with everything I would need, the tools and resources, to make it happen. He put me to the test, and I came out of a very difficult situation victorious. I try to see God and the good in everything. It's so easy for the devil to point out the bad, but the devil just comes to kill and destroy. So if that's his mission, he doesn't like marriage because marriage is a godly thing. Marriage is under attack.

Of course, none of us is perfect, and we all have most certainly done something to the other. But should we allow the devil to sneak in and attack us in our most vulnerable places? Our marriage should be a place of safety, comfort, and happiness. While temptations surround each of us every day and from every side, we do not have to succumb to those temptations, valuing what we have more than any possibility of temporary fulfillment. The cost is too high, and the game of Russian roulette is too dangerous to play with temptation.

Life is about valuing your feelings and your own life. I am my daughters' first example of womanhood and what strength is. I know that the alignment in my life could drastically change something in their lives, and I am responsible for doing what I can for them. While I may not know until they are grown the impact that my decisions have had on them, I know that today they are happy, healthy, and know they are loved.

What are your goals for your children?

____

____

____

____

____

____

____

____

"Behold, I send you out as sheep in the midst of wolves. Therefore be wise as serpents and harmless as doves." Matthew 10:16 NKJV

God said that if you are going to pray, don't worry; if you are going to worry, don't pray. I had to fall on my face a couple of times because I had to do what was right for me and these kids. I had been comfortable, and now, on my own, I was being stretched. But God!

As He always does, He provided. God came through as my husband began stripping away the financial support, always meeting our needs. This was during the pandemic, so the federal stimulus checks were right on time. I picked up another job to make ends meet. It made me question: had I been so dependent on my husband that I didn't hear God all the time? I didn't see God all the time? And therefore, I didn't go to God all the time? Is that why He removed the person from my life so I could get closer to and depend on Him?

Of course, I had been going to church and was still very faithful, but did I one hundred percent depend on God? Maybe He needed to remind me where my help comes from. Was I not being as good a daughter as I thought I was or as I was to my husband? I had always had a relationship with God but felt a shift. When you move stability out of the way, where do we turn? Pointing fingers at the other person is easy, and I could easily throw stones at my husband for all his wrongs. But where is my accountability in this?

I was now a single mother and immediately jumped into survival mode; the daily routine of the house, getting the girls to counseling, and frankly, operating in faith. I just knew that a better day was going to come. I began to get up at 5 am to pray. I had to tap into the strength God had instilled in me in a new way, so I learned how to meditate, making me feel more self-aware and stronger.

My main focus was on the girls, and I had neglected to check on myself. In fact, I was so overprotective of their feelings and emotions about the situation that I didn't realize they were fine. Truly fine! Ultimately, I learned they had known their father was stepping out even before I suspected it. Children watch our every move and instinctively knew something was wrong. Hovering over my cubs, I failed to see my new reality had been right in front of my eyes.

Of course, this was a huge adjustment for me, especially when I was used to looking to the left and right, leaning on another person to make decisions with, no matter how large or small those decisions were. We were a team and discussed everything about what was good for the family unit.

We had several businesses together during our marriage, including a catering service. I was already an author, brought women together at a shelter, and had been on television and radio. I was well into making a name for myself with my husband by my side. So when my marriage came tumbling down in my face, so did my image.

I had worn being a wife and a mom like a badge of honor, with the other things falling closely behind. The divorce robbed me of the business part of life. It took my voice and my name, and I started turning down opportunities as they arose. I felt ashamed that I was now divorced. I was hiding behind the pandemic as an excuse for not speaking on stages, but in reality, it was just a way to hide behind how I truly felt. I was uncomfortable talking about my marriage not working out because no one signs up to get divorced. Although it is not the same as death, I still grieved the loss of my marriage and had to navigate those complicated feelings and emotions as if someone close to me had died.

Although I mentioned previously that I had suspected him of being unfaithful and my daughters confirmed it later, the infidelity did not break us apart. I had told him I would leave if he did it again, but ultimately, his indiscretions were forgivable. I am not saying that it was okay or that people should go out and cheat! I am saying that everyone has a different breaking point; mine was abandonment.

In my eyes, what had I done (or not done) that would make him pack up all of his belongings and leave? What about our home was not good enough for him? How could we reconcile his abandoning the house where we were raising our daughters? Our home was now changed, and the dynamics would never be the same with or without him. The cost of his return was too great, and I was unwilling to do it. I was unwilling to compromise who I was or lose Lillie altogether. Besides, who would I be as a mother if I compromised myself? I held him to a higher standard, placing him on a pedestal as I felt warranted for his profession and his being. He fell from this position the moment he walked out that door.

I have always been active on social media and throughout my many networks. My life suddenly shifted so profoundly that I shied away from posting or attending the many events I was used to. I was not ready to answer the questions that people undoubtedly had or the shocked look on their faces when I shared that we were divorced. I decided to keep my married name, "Smith," for my girls, although I ultimately know that my ex does not deserve me keeping his name. A friend talked me out of changing my name back to "Simmons," but Simmons was who I had become again at this stage, and I didn't need Smith.

I was still worried about the girls' well-being and their perspective of their father. He does not come around, and they barely have a relationship with him. No matter how one becomes a single mother, I expect many women are faced with the tough questions and, more importantly, providing answers to their children as to 'why.' I didn't have the answers for them then, nor do I have more answers for them now, even after counseling. I believe many of their questions should be directed at their father for him to answer.

It took a while for me to realize that I was doing all of this on my own. This transition from 'Smith' to 'Simmons' knocked me to my knees because I thought I had something altogether. But I didn't! It was not what I thought it was. Have you ever put together a large puzzle and get to the last few pieces, only to realize that the corner puzzle piece is a tiny bit different than you thought and no longer fits inside the image? Oh, how it disrupts *everything*!

I still could not reconcile this man who was now neglecting his daughters and the man who I married. It was like a switch had suddenly been turned off, and he no longer cared. It makes me question whether I ever knew him at all. Is it possible that I married someone like that? Sadly, I may never get the closure or the answers the girls and I are looking for.

Now, as a single mother and divorcee, I am relearning and understanding who I am. When you become a wife and mother, naturally, everyone's needs seem to come before your own. I am now working on loving *me* for who I am and who I have been created to be.

I am learning about myself as a thirty-something instead of the teenager who met her future husband. My mindset and perspectives have changed, and I am mindful that although I may not be someone's wife, I am someone's mom (times two). I wear that hat with pride, knowing that in an instant, a title or a position can change. I have witnessed it firsthand. But knowing myself and loving myself unapologetically is one thing no one can take away from me. As women, we cater so much to others, not realizing that we lose a little bit of ourselves each time we do not experience the same in return.

Thankfully, although I feel so much was stolen from me by my husband's decision to leave, the one thing that could not be taken was my womanhood—my confidence in the woman I am. Just because I saw something as valuable does not mean it was valued the same way. I stood on my truth once he decided to leave, and I don't regret where life has taken me.

What are you standing on?

____

____

____

____

____

____

____

____

"Trust in the Lord with all your heart, And lean not on your own understanding." Proverbs 3:5 NKJV

I am now standing on my own and returning to who I was before I was married. There are no second guesses. There is no reason for me to look to the left or the right, listening for another person's opinion. I'm now uncomfortable standing on my own. Going through a divorce where the husband was so involved and to a place where he is no longer involved is a big step. I think I took for granted all he had done because I was just going through life. Now I had no one to rely on for the big decisions, the impactful purchases, and the forward-thinking choices but myself. I had to rely on only what I knew from living on my own before getting married and the maturity I had gained while I was married.

There was no help. Every game, cheerleading practice, or counseling session would be done on my own. After navigating life alone for about a year, as Marie, I realized that "I've got this." The girls and I had created a structure in our household that we were growing accustomed to. I had to be comfortable in my final decisions with the girls since I had no one to bounce ideas and thoughts off of. Now I was doing it all by myself. I had done life before on my own, but it was different now with two girls, so I had to handle life from a different perspective.

As adversity tends to do when we are faced with it, I began to see a change in myself. I was changing into a more grown version of myself. I used to discuss everything with my partner related to our daughters and what was best for them; now, the only one I could converse with was God. Although I normally pray about everything, I took to sitting on my own, asking Him about the best course of action or the right way of handling something. I had to press in and lean on God for everything. Everything that I knew about myself was being tested and stretched. Some days were more difficult than others; I would cry, wail, and moan. There were days when I would want to engage with people and others when I needed to be alone, sitting in God's presence. No matter what life was throwing at me, I always showed my authentic self to my girls, the many sides to me as a woman; the vulnerable side, the passionate and loving side, and even the confused and struggling side. But it was more important for me to demonstrate how to handle each of these scenarios and all that life would throw at them. I taught them how to meditate, to grab hold of the idea that they could do whatever they needed no matter what. The devil comes to steal, kill, and destroy, but I wanted to show them that you can overcome anything he brings.

It is all about how you view things, your perspective. A better day is coming, although today may seem dark and dismal. My transition back to Marie, the woman I was before, was slow, often painful, but surprisingly necessary. It was an awakening that I could evolve, grow, and learn by detaching myself from those things that kept me comfortable. I had to adapt to being a single woman again.

It was during this time that I met a new friend. As I was growing, he was there, gently pushing me to be the best version of myself from afar. I had been so used to my husband being there every day, as married couples are, that I needed to ensure I had space to handle my business. I wanted to think and do things for myself, but he was there to pick me up when I stumbled. As God does, He gives us exactly what we need when we need it, and I believe He placed this man in my life at the right time for the right purpose. Ironically, I met him two weeks after my husband walked out on us.

Now, from the outside, because of the timing, it may seem that I was already involved with this man, my friend, while I was married. But others may fail to see that I was so committed to my relationship and marriage that I would never have even considered a friendship with another man other than my husband. I would never have given another man even a sideways glance because I did not want that type of energy in my marriage. Again, God has His way of knowing when the timing is right!

Meeting my friend was part of my transformation or restoration of Marie, the new and improved version. My husband had been my knight in shining armor, so I had never envisioned myself in this position, pushing through life alone, nor could I see myself with another man. But I believe that nothing just happens; the divorce, my renewal, and my return to Marie were part of God's plan all along. No matter how uncomfortable we become in situations or how painful, we must go through it because God knows that there is more and better waiting for us on the other side. What I thought was my knight, my complete, my period, was actually a comma in the story of my life.

At this point, walking through life in survival mode with open wounds, searching for direction, my friend was a breath of fresh air. He would get up every morning at 5 am and call me just to pray with me. We never missed a day of prayer. He did not want anything from me but simply to pray, and when we were finished, he would politely say, "Have a nice day," before ending the call.

I had blinders on as I simply put one foot in front of the other each day and could not see how God was orchestrating everything. Of course, I was still giving Him the glory every day, thanking Him for waking me and allowing my day to go smoothly. But I could not see how everything that was happening around me was for the greater good, for *my* greater good.

We often forget to thank God for every little thing that He does. Have you ever stopped to thank God for waking you up 5 minutes late? Maybe that happened because He was orchestrating life so that you would avoid the accident or that thing that would harm you or your children. When you start going through life, its ups and downs, challenges and joys, when you sit back and start to smell the roses, or in my case, the Lillies, you will realize how truly blessed you are and give thanks. That's where my blessings come from. That's where the overflow comes from. God came to give you life and give you life more abundantly, but it doesn't say anywhere that you are not going to go through anything in the meantime.

I had made a life with my husband, and although we lived abundantly, I was comfortable. I could not at the time be thankful for all that He had saved me from. I could not see that there was so much more to life or to Marie. That life is gone, and I am now comfortable living as Marie, standing on my own two feet, calling all the shots myself, unapologetically raising my daughters. Whether my ex-husband stands with us or not, we are still moving forward. Of course, they still cry and have a lot of questions. Although I am the scorned wife, he is still their father. I do not bash or belittle him, but I always tell them the truth unapologetically if they ask me questions. My job as their parent is to provide clarity from my point of view.

Marie has returned, and although she was always there, hanging back, she always put everyone else's needs before her own. Becoming a wife and mother at such a young age, I didn't realize the true principles of life. I was so busy checking the boxes; wife – check, mother – check, everyone is good – check. I didn't realize that the true glory was in the One providing all this for me. A higher power was doing all of this, and it was definitely not me or my husband.

He wasn't my night in shining armor because it was not how it was supposed to be. That's how I viewed him, but he didn't view himself that way, and I couldn't change that. But so many women stay for so long trying to change their spouse. But in the midst of it, you lose who the hell you are because you are trying to prove something that you'll never be able to prove to that individual because that's a personal attack on them. That's something that they have to go through. Seek counseling, seek God, fall on their face, cry it out; that's something they must deal with.

But I don't think a lot of us are taught enough that when things are a hundred percent ugly, call it out as a hundred percent ugly. Don't sit here and try to make something fit that isn't fitting. Have you ever spoken to a couple who has been married for, let's say, 40 or 50 years? They may say, "It's been great." But has it been great the entire time? Sure, maybe in the beginning or now, but what about all the stuff in between? I want to encourage women to take a different approach. I am not telling women not to get married but to get married without losing their individuality. We all say that we will not lose ourselves when we join our spouse in marriage, but it is easy to do. As long as we're comfortable and trust our husband enough, we will follow his lead naturally. It just happens.

Even several years after the divorce, and as they grow and mature, my daughters still ask me many questions about their father. Why don't we hear from dad more? Why does he rush me off the phone? Why doesn't he come around more often? As my youngest says, "That's not my dad." I was so happy to hear her say that because the person we see now is not the same man I married. The type of guy I married loved, he provided, protected, and honored. The man that we see now is destructive and has no concern for what he says or who he hurts with his actions. I would never marry a guy like that, let alone have a child with a man like that. If the man I married were still around, we would still be friends today, and my children would have their father in their lives. We would still be co-parenting our daughters because that is the type of man he had always shown me to be; respectful, honorable, and just a stand-up guy. But this person, I don't know who this man is, and frankly, had this man shown up when we first met, I would have run the other way.

However, let's look at this from another perspective. Maybe he had to turn into this type of person to make room for the one to come behind. In the spiritual realm, he had to change so God could get my undivided attention because everything happens for a reason, and it is already written. He had to change so I could move on from him to what was destined to be mine. God had more for me, but if my ex-husband had not changed, my growth would have been hindered. God removed the distraction because I was so comfortable with and accustomed to that life that I could not receive or even see all God had in store for me. He said, "Let me make sure it is all ugly so you can return to where you need to be and go further. And when you go further, you will touch so many more lives." What did God mean?

So I could speak more. I could tell more people about Him. I could show people how my life has changed because of my relationship with God. Praying and worrying don't go together. God showed me that I could not do both. Just because my husband left did not mean my whole life would stop.

Marie has come a long way and mentally has grown a lot. Growth begins by changing the subconscious mind. Although it hurt like hell, I know that all I experienced was meant for me. Of course, no one goes into a marriage to get divorced. Nobody wants to go through the pain of missing your loved one and certainly not being ugly with each other after you have taken a vow to love one another. I had given my ex-husband all of myself, changed my body, and given him two children. I certainly never planned or imagined life would turn out as it did. Each time he tried to come back to reconcile with me, I kept pushing for the divorce. Once I realized that enough was enough, there was no turning back. I knew that proceeding down this path would cost me something—pain, heartache, financial ruin. But the reward of setting the example for my girls and reclaiming the Marie that had been buried for so long made it all worth it.

But God had other plans.

As Marie reemerged and came into her power, I realized things had to change. I was comfortable, but now I am developing transferable skills I can pass along to my girls. Life lessons that I can instill in them. The resilience can be used in any life situation; careers end, jobs can be lost, and relationships die, but you have to have resilience on the inside of you to see that there is life after rejection; there is life after loss; there is life after betrayal. There is power in going through troubles and challenges because you come back stronger and with more clarity.

Marie was trying to do it on her own. Marie didn't have the village, or that is how I felt. I had been so used to my ex and I doing everything; now it was just me. I didn't think I could turn to anyone to replace the help I had lost. I felt like I was on an island; I know I was not, but my mind had convinced me of that.

Who is your village?

____

____

Lillie

"Fear not, for I have redeemed you; I have called you by your name; You are Mine. When you pass through the waters, I will be with you; And through the rivers, they shall not overflow you. When you walk through the fire, you shall not be burned, Nor shall the flame scorch you." Isaiah 43: 1-2 NKJV

October 4th, 2022. Lillie woke up on the floor in excruciating pain and was rushed to the hospital. I had a cyst sitting on my right ovary, which was 26 centimeters, equal to 10 inches. While the doctor told me it could be cancer due to its size, I firmly and adamantly declared that the devil is a liar! You can't worry and pray in the same space, so I just put it in the hands of my faithful prayer warriors. I knew I needed enough strength to get through the surgery, and worry would sap my energy and will. Laying there worrying would not have done me any good, so I focused on raising my girls and how I needed to be healthy and strong for them.

I was gaining my independence and just getting adjusted to being a single mom, being by myself and doing things on my own, and then suddenly, I was fighting for my life in a different way. Right before my eyes, I saw the fruits of my parenting as my young daughters witnessed their mother writhing in pain yet had the wherewithal to call 911 and calmly walk the operator through the situation. There was nothing that I could do. I was conscious but was in so much pain that I could not be of assistance to anyone.

As I lay there in my hospital bed, my new man by my side, I experienced a new kind of love and appreciation. His patience, understanding, and kindness were endless and oozed from every pore. The Lord knows anyone must be patient when another is going through a storm, and at the time, I didn't see it for what it was—LOVE! His faith was boundless and supported me when mine wavered.

Had the circumstances been different, my ex-husband would have been there because he was married to me. But when someone truly cares for you and loves you enough to do whatever it takes, the love is palpable. Although I thought I had experienced love, that love was demonstrated at another level. I believed I had a connection, but God pulled back the covers to expose a higher, more profound connection. And my girls got to experience the love of a father without the presence of their biological father. I had never been loved like that before. If you allow yourself to let go of what you feel is normal, you will experience blessings like you never thought possible.

The life I had in my old book was my normal; now, *this* is my new normal. For anyone scared about what lies ahead, trust me when I say that you will not know what is waiting for you until you let go. When you allow your bubble of what you know as normal to be busted, you will create and experience a new bubble filled with love, joy, and fulfillment.

In my brokenness, I was not able to see love—true love!

The old me had to die, nearly literally, for the new one to understand and wrap my mind around the idea that life is limitless. It was not in God's plan for me to die physically that day because He had bigger plans for me.

We often get stuck in what we created as normal, afraid to step out to see what is on the other side. When pushed, what I found was new love. I have a better relationship with my girls because I now see them in a different light and have a new respect for them. As parents, we want to save our children from harm or hurt, but when your kids turn around and save you, that takes the relationship to a higher level of respect. When faced with a crisis, their maturity created a new unbreakable bond between us.

As independent as Marie was becoming, Lillie was quickly reminded that it takes a village and a strong support system. I didn't have to do it on my own. The devil saw what I was doing and tried to take me out, make me think I couldn't do it, or test my will. But what he doesn't know is that his test only made my faith in God and myself that much stronger.

Lying in that bed, praying for my healing, I heard God say, "It's already written for you," and I knew. I knew that with His hand on my life, I could fight against the image of what I thought others saw of Lillie. Regardless of what happened with my ex-husband, God already knew it was in His plan for my life, and I could not fight against what was written. I could only get up and continue to move forward. Even though in those tough moments I felt like giving up, there was more for me. I had to open my hand and let go to let God. All that I had been through gave me strength and a voice.

When my ex-husband stepped away, it was more like he had passed away than simply walked out. This type of man that I was married to was an all-in type of guy. We had a partnership where we shared everything, from responsibilities to chores to cooking and caring for our children. So, when he left and took all of that with him, it left a gaping hole I now had to fill—just me!

But now Lillie is moving up, out, and beyond! She is restored, whole, and new! I am no longer in a position or relationship where I have to dim my light. I know that not everyone will understand or be able to relate. Consider this: Have you ever had a woman comment on your parenting style, but she has no children? What about the parent who wants to advise you on raising three or four children, yet she only has one? For some, it may make more sense when you get married, but for now, understand that although Lillie's light was not dimmed, it was certainly different. I want to simply remind everyone and hope you will remember as you build your relationship to remain true to yourself while creating a life with your spouse and family. You may not be able to understand that type of relationship, the one in which you are true partners, if you have never experienced it.

I know that I have been blessed. The house, the cars, the money, the career, whatever someone else may strive to have, I experienced it. However, with that experience comes a great deal of responsibility, especially in passing along what I have learned to others. With my story, I hope the light bulb turns off for certain people and the wisdom kicks in.

Of course, no relationship is a hundred percent. Unfortunately, many people will gamble with their relationships, searching for whatever they believe is missing. You don't play Russian roulette with true love. Sadly, my ex-husband was willing to place that bet, and he lost.

Now, Lillie, who has proven that she is like the flower, the Lilly of the Valley, withstanding every storm, is firmly planted and seeking the sun's warmth. As she stretches her arms toward all she has ever dreamed, she knows that with God, she will continue to move forward. Having overcome so much, she received a clean slate on which she will write her story. She brings her dignity, morals, and respect into her next relationship. As Maya Angelou said, "once someone shows you who they are, you better believe them." Once her ex-husband revealed his true character, Lillie was no longer willing to compromise herself, no matter how painful it was. She is watering good seeds through her businesses, charitable organization, and mentoring. God has big plans for Lillie, and she is swaying in the wind as God breathes new life into her circumstances according to His plan.

Everything happens for a reason. Although I was concerned about bringing another man into our home, trying to replace their father's presence, my new friend, who I can now lovingly call my boyfriend, came in and has never left their side. When one foot stepped out, the other foot stepped in. I was holding my girls back from something so beautiful—a healthy relationship with a male figure. In such a short amount of time, he was able to develop a relationship and show them so much love as if he were there all the time. It was a sign from God; from the outside, no one would even know that he is not their father.

It is amazing to see the blossom of my life bloom as I release those things I've been holding onto. Even though I had been through something so ugly, I was able to find something so beautiful. Once you open your hand and release stuff, stop trying to hold onto it; amazing gifts will flow in and out of your hand. Focus on what's in front of you; sometimes, love is right there, and we don't even realize it.

Nothing can get in when you ball your fist, trying to hold tight to what you once had. But if you open up your hand and allow stuff to flow in and out, if it's real, it will stick. If something is no longer good for you, you must let it go. In my ex-husband's case, I loved him enough to let him go. Now did I think I would turn into all of this? This amazing version of myself? No, but it was necessary. Maybe I wouldn't appreciate another guy the way I appreciate this man, who brings loyalty, communication, and understanding.

When you look back at what you were holding onto, you realize that what you thought was a lack of time was really excuses. When you are comfortable in your life and your world, you neglect to see where you are not being fulfilled or satisfied. Your vision is clouded to the changes that have occurred within yourself and the loss of self you have experienced. You no longer apply pressure on yourself to continue to grow and develop, denying yourself access to all that awaits you.

Stop getting caught up in the fairy tale and see things for what they are. If my ex had been an awesome father when we were married, he should still be an awesome father now that we're divorced. If he had been a good friend while we were married, he would still be a good friend now that we're divorced because we shared so much; that bond should always be there. On the other hand, don't stay with someone because it looks good on paper. You deserve you!

As a woman, we can't raise a man to be a man, but we can raise them to be husbands because we know what we want. Mothers, raise up your men to be good to their wives. Encourage them to walk in their purpose and shine their light.

Refo life, rebuild, start over

I can overcome anything

Walking by faith and not by sight

Being positive

Loving self

Walking in my purpose

Unapologetically that's me

Life is a journey. You never know what you're going to get from it. However, enjoy the ride and be happy with all your decisions or choices that you have made.

Are you ready?

____

____

____

____

____

____

____

41

"I Battle Alone"

It was bought to my attention that I don't smile,
Well true enough it has been awhile;

These past two years have been a lot of ups and
downs,

I have developed PTSD to certain sounds;

There's a Battle within every day,

To where it's just easier to say I'm okay;

God didn't give me the spirit of fear,

So my prayer has been to open my eyes and my
ears;(to be able to see and hear God's plans for my
life)

I want to be made whole,

But I've been hurt and the pain so deep it's
attached to my soul;

The moment I heard ashes to ashes and dust to
dirt,

All that did was amplified my hurt;

Then the devil tries to be slick,

Try to distract me with his bags of tricks;

But little do he know I might be in a daze,

But he can't have my praise;

I know without my praise it can cause delays,

I don't care how many doors seem to be closed I will praise him anyway;(up and down the hallway)

All I need is that one open door with my name on it,

I will walk through boldly, anointed, appointed, with the authority from God and any other way he sees fit;

Dawn has been broken to the core,

But her faith is in God she knows he has something in store;

As I wait on God promises,

To be honest In my subconscious;

I flashback to prophecies and prayers,

All I can do is work on me and prepare;

I know the calling on my life is great and mighty,

The reason why the devil constantly tries to fight me;

But I remind him that I'm a fighter and a daughter of a King,

I will win this fight in or out the ring;

I am going to endure until the end,

I might be broken now but I know a potter that's reconstructing me again;

I'm trusting this process choosing to Battle Alone and there's no hard feelings,

It's through God's way I will receive my complete healing;

There's nothing I need for anyone to do or say,

But the most helpful thing you can do is pray;

There's a void that only God can fill,

And prayer is the only way I know how to deal;

~ I Battle Alone ~ God's strength □ □

Book: *The Battle Before Dawn*

Email address:
Lifeunderpressurepodcast@post.com

Website:
https://wisdom.app/renewedstrength5/ask

Acknowledgment

To my Father in Heaven for ordering my steps with your mercy and grace. I'm humbly thankful.

I want to acknowledge the extraordinary debt I owe my village, which has been there for all my ups and downs. Thank you for providing your shoulders, time, words of wisdom, and, most importantly, your prayers. I elevate to new levels because of my family, friends, and my sisterhood.

Laylah and Lyric, you both are the best of me. Never forget "once you know it, no one can take it away from you." Be YOU. Never let anyone stop you from being YOU!

A special thank you to Rachel for being my rock throughout this writing journey. I appreciate you for your time.

To my future husband, thank you for walking down this journey of healing with me, never letting my hand go, and never letting me hold my head down during the hard days. For always uplifting me, pushing, praying, and being there. Always reminding me that I'm a Queen! Your Queen . . . I'm so open to our future with you and the boys!

A special thank you to my son, who came to me as a stepson.

Reginald A Smith Jr

I love you so much. Your smile brightens my world. Thanking God for your life every day!

Thank you for never allowing anyone to stop you from being my son. Thank you for always looking at me and treating me like your mom.

Or, in your words, "MA."

Know that you are on a journey of transformation. You are exploring the wisdom of your soul. You are shedding old beliefs and stories that no longer fit who you are becoming. Stay strong! Be brave! Be YOU!

Thank you, Son! I love you unapologetically!

This book is dedicated to my granny Jessie Thompson and my mother, Dorothy Griffin. Thank you both for being a part of my life; you two are some strong women!

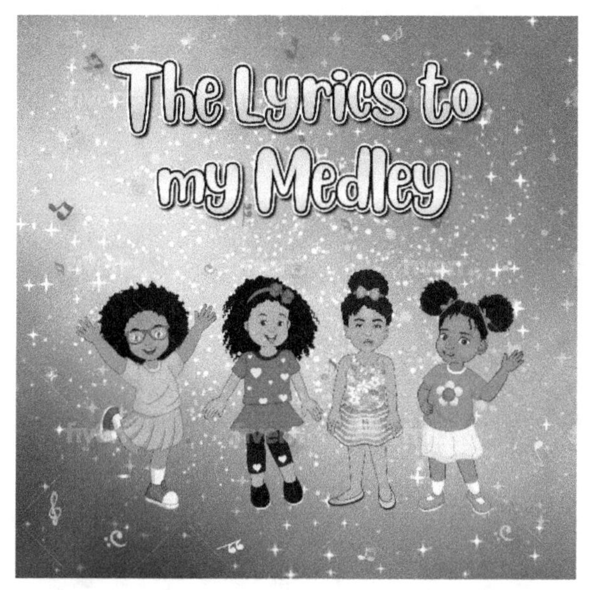

Stay on the lookout for two more great books!

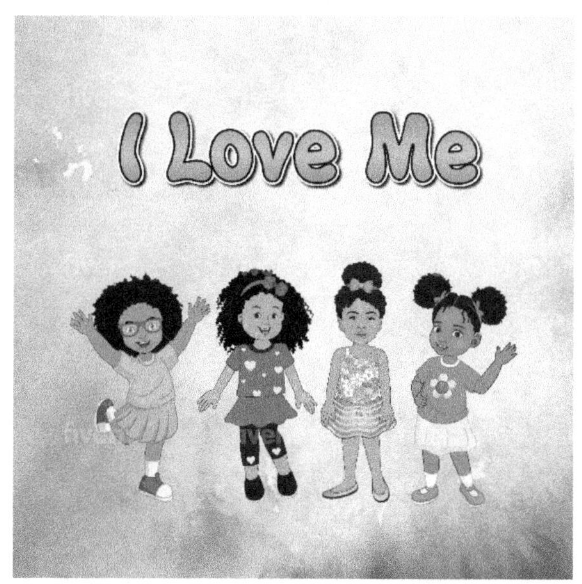